The Miracle Ball Method

The Miracle

relieve your pain
reshape your body
reduce your stress

Ball Method

by **Elaine Petrone**

Workman Publishing, New York

Copyright © 2003 by Elaine Petrone

Library of Congress Cataloging-in-Publication Data

Petrone, Elaine.
The miracle ball method: relieve your pain, reshape your body,
reduce your stress / by Elaine Petrone.
p. cm.
ISBN 978-0-7611-2868-7
1. Backache–Exercise therapy. 2. Pain–Exercise therapy. 3. Stress relaxation.
4. Physical fitness. I. Title.
RD771.B217P475 2003
617.5'64062–dc22   2003062136

Workman books are available at special discounts when purchased in bulk for premiums and sales promotions as well as for fund-raising or educational use. Special editions can also be created to specification. For details, contact the Special Sales Director at the address below or send an email to specialmarkets@workman.com.

Design by Paul Hanson and Elizabeth Johnsboen

Workman Publishing Company, Inc.
225 Varick Street
New York, NY 10014-4381
workman.com

WORKMAN is a registered trademark of Workman Publishing Co., Inc.

Printed in China
First printing December 2003
30

*Dedicated to the memories of Chris
and Mary Curas, and Paula Curas Didelot*

Contents

PART ONE

The Basics

PART TWO

On the Ball

Foreword

I have known Elaine Petrone for more than ten years now. She has worked with my patients in the rehabilitation center where I practice. Her method of ball therapy gives people the tools to help themselves feel better. Many of my patients are struggling with such chronic conditions as back pain, fibromyalgia, unhealed injury, arthritis, as well as physiological reactions to stress. Elaine's method gives them ways of reducing their bodies' stress and relieving their pain. I highly recommend *The Miracle Ball Method,* as so many of my patients have received relief from it.

The special needs limitations, and responses of each individual cannot be anticipated. The Miracle Ball Method is not intended for the purpose of diagnosing or as a substitute for medical treatment.

Introduction

Welcome to *The Miracle Ball Method*. You may be reading this book because you have chronic pain for which you are seeking relief. You may have come to it because you feel overwhelmed by stress. Or you may have realized that there are certain parts of your body that no longer feel as toned as they should and that you are looking older and tired as a result. Whatever brings you here, whether it is the nagging pain of a back injury, say, or the intense stress that you may be under, or just a general desire to look good, the solution to relieving your pain and stress is the same: it is to reduce your muscle tension.

The Cycle of Pain

Excess muscle tension can come from three sources: an injury, such as a car or sports accident; stress, including the ordinary rigors of family life or financial troubles (even good things—planning a wedding or having a baby—can bring stress); and alignment problems, such as scoliosis or just poor posture. Any one of these things may have caused your tension, or your suffering may have a combination of causes. No matter what the origin, your muscles respond to stress by activating a cycle of pain in your body. For instance, back pain may affect not only the muscles surrounding your spine, but those at your neck, hips, and other areas. It's a vicious cycle. You feel stress or experience an injury, say, so your muscles tighten, and when your muscles tighten the result is poor breathing habits, which results in higher stress levels, which cause your muscles to tighten further. The cycle is hard to break unless you can find a way to release the tension in your overworked muscles.

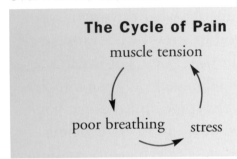

The Cycle of Pain

muscle tension

poor breathing   stress

When muscles become tense and imbalanced, your body's natural correct alignment system cannot work properly. Furthermore, muscles that remain tense for long periods lose the ability to relax at all, resulting in chronic pain. The best way to illustrate this is to imagine holding a tennis ball in your hand. Imagine gripping the tennis ball as tightly as you can for five hours—or even five days. Can you imagine how awful the pain would be? Can you imagine how much you would want to let go of it? But even if you did finally relax your hand, what would happen? It would remain curved in a claw shape for some time. It would probably take hours for the hand to relax into its normal state. Many of us are holding so much tension in our bodies that, despite intense pain, we are unable to relax the muscles: Our bodies have forgotten how.

There are many books on the market that are designed to help you alleviate stress and pain. Some require physical effort, such as stretching. Others suggest meditation or other mental techniques. My method is the simplest one I've found for relieving pain, reducing stress, and in the process, reshaping your body. It starts with what I call your body formula:

Your Body Formula
Weight + Breathing = Release of Tension

I have found that if you breathe fully while allowing yourself to feel the weight of your body, you enable your muscles to relax and you experience immense relief. Loosening your muscles enables your body to realign, and when your muscles are limber and your skeleton is properly aligned, you do not experience pain.

The actual method is simple: You place your weight on the balls and feel your body give in to them. You breathe fully to bring oxygen to your muscles, which in turn restores feeling to them. Because most of us chronically breathe only with our upper chests, our muscles are stiff and as a result we hold ourselves rigidly. When muscles are rigid you have less feeling in them. You can't move what you don't feel, so when muscles are clenched and tight, they resist gravity. (For example, when you are stuck in traffic your shoulders clench upward toward your ears—as you tighten them, they rise and resist gravity.) In order to release those muscles you must be able to feel them first, which breathing will help you do, then feel their weight. The body is supported by the ball, the muscles release their tension, and the pain disappears. This may happen immediately or it may come gradually over time; each person's experience is unique. But every person who has followed my method has experienced immense relief. *You simply cannot help but get results when you reduce your muscle tension.*

In addition to pain relief, my program has two important side effects: relief from anxiety and the reshaping of your entire body. It is difficult to feel stressed when the symptoms of stress—clenched muscles and shallow breathing—are removed. And you may be surprised at the effect my method has on your figure. Tight muscles are thick and stiff; relaxed muscles are long and flexible. Would you rather have short, thick muscles or long, supple ones surrounding your waist, abdomen, and thighs?

In addition to delivering results, my method of ball therapy is easy to do—deceptively easy. Visualization, meditation, biofeedback, and behavioral therapy all require too much effort for my liking. When I tried these and other mind-over-body methods, I always found that my mind was too active and that it was a struggle—and a contradiction in terms—to "try" to relax my mind. It was too much work for me. What I needed to relax, it seemed to me, was not my mind but my body. Now I don't worry about what my mind is doing. I just get on the balls, breathe, and let my body do the rest.

My Story

I understand the feelings of my students because I have had my own experience with chronic pain. I understand the anxiety and questions it can produce: Why is this happening? Why can't I find help? And why is it affecting so many other parts of my life? I developed my method of ball therapy in response to my need to find answers to these questions and to heal my own body.

When I first started having back pain, I assumed it would be temporary and go away on its own over time. I was in college and studying to be a dancer, practicing four hours a day, seven days a week. I believed I was going to get rid of that back pain and move on. I was wrong. The pain got worse. It seemed to come out of nowhere, and it began to affect not only my back, but my right leg as well.

I visited doctors, but nobody could give me a satisfactory explanation or tell me what could be done to make things right. My general practitioner assured me that it was just a pulled muscle and I would be fine. A chiropractor took X rays, diagnosed it as a pinched nerve, and tried to realign me. All the treatments I tried—

massage therapy, various movement techniques, shiatsu, diet cures—worked only temporarily. The pain worsened and eventually I was unable to dance at all.

I was devastated. As time went by I developed symptoms of post-traumatic stress syndrome: I had panic and anxiety attacks; I became agoraphobic. My body was overstressed and fatigued as I fought the depression that was overtaking me. I woke up with night sweats, with parts of my body numb. A constant burning radiated from the palm of my right hand, up my arm, across my chest, and down the other arm. I took tranquilizers to ease my anxiety and pain relievers to ease my physical pain.

I was looking for a diagnosis—any diagnosis—because in my mind, if an ailment could be diagnosed, then surely a cure existed or could be found. My doctors did what they could, telling me they had ruled out any major diseases, offering sympathy, and all of them making sure I understood that my injury was not going to be healed easily, if at all. In the end there was no diagnosis, and I was told, "You should consider yourself lucky if you can walk without a limp, and you should forget ever dancing again." Within several months my right leg had withered to half the size of my left. At this point I became desperate and started asking anybody and everybody if they knew of something—anything— I could try to heal my leg.

I found a handful of teachers in New York City who worked differently from the experts I had seen. Most doctors told me to stop moving; these teachers told me to keep moving. They told me my injury wasn't about a weakness; it was about excess muscle tension. The amount of effort I was

using to try to heal myself was interfering
with my body's own alignment system. I
found teachers who worked with balls,
then I found teachers who worked with
breathing and alignment in new ways. I
started listening intently to dance teachers
who spoke about using and shifting the
weight of your body as you moved. I started
reading research about reducing tension by
tensing muscles and then letting go. I
learned at least a little something from
everyone I visited and from everything
I read, and the pieces began to come
together. I started to realize that I had been

taking the wrong approach. I was searching for some activity, some movement to rid myself of aches and pains. But I was overlooking the body's own ability to realign itself using little more than gravity. And I understood that it wasn't a method that was just for my own body: it was a method for everyone's body.

I experimented with the balls, which I placed under different parts of my body to see what happened. To my shock, I learned that by doing less—by doing absolutely nothing, actually—and by simply giving in to the balls, my body realigned. I was delighted and amazed. How could doing nothing bring such dramatic results? I was thrilled to be recovering, so I used my balls constantly, spending four to six hours daily resting on a ball, releasing my muscles, letting myself go. When I wasn't on the ball, I was starting to dance again, and I was looking and feeling better than I had in years.

I never thought I would devote my life to teaching this method, but my friends and colleagues became curious about how I had healed myself. I was approached by people in pain—"I have a problem with my back, I have terrible headaches, I have a knee injury. Can you help?"—and my method always alleviated their pain. Eventually, the word got to friends who were doctors who invited me to consult with some of their toughest patients. I had no idea that there were so many people who had very similar experiences with chronic pain and anxiety, from crippling back pain to severe panic attacks. Now I teach my method to other professionals, including physical therapists, personal trainers, and massage therapists, in addition to teaching students of my own in settings from gyms to hospitals.

I sincerely hope that this book offers you the relief you seek. Please feel free to contact me if you have questions or feedback as you work. Visit my Web site, www.elainepetrone.com or e-mail me at elaine@elainepetrone.com.

PART ONE

The Basics

CHAPTER ONE

How to Use this Book

You can start this program today. There is no special equipment you need to buy, no special outfit you need to wear, no special time for doing the exercises. You just need a patch of floor and the balls that come with the book. I do recommend that you wear comfortable clothes, avoiding tight waistbands or straps.

But in a pinch, I have even done these exercises in jeans (unbuttoned for comfort).

About the Ball

There are many types of balls for exercise and physical therapy: hard balls, medicine balls, large physiotherapy balls, and tennis balls, to mention only a few. The Miracle Ball is different. I designed it with two things in mind: the perfect amount of give and the right size. You can feel the weight of your body while you rest on it, but I've made sure that it is still small enough and yielding enough so that you won't have to strain or struggle to stay on it. The ball is just a tool to help you feel the weight of your body. You don't need to push against it, rub against it, slide all over it, or attempt to make it do something. The ball is there for you to sink into. Your goal is to allow your body to heal itself, de-stress, and return to its natural alignment. All you have to do is breathe and feel your weight. It's that simple. Your body will do the rest.

These balls are incredibly tough and easy to care for. They are designed for every student, no matter the body type, and should last for years. If your balls get dirty, simply wipe them with a damp cloth and dry them off. If you feel that they are deflating too much, you can add air with an old fashioned bike pump.

Here is how I recommend you follow the program: Find a comfortable spot in your home. You'll be lying on the floor, so use a place that has carpeting or an exercise mat or quilt. Try to find a spot that's warm so that you will be comfortable and able to relax completely. Turn the phone off and keep the balls on the floor near you. If you will need to answer the telephone, keep it within reach. If you want to watch TV while you work, turn it on and keep the remote control handy. (I don't recommend watching TV on your first few times working with the balls because I'd like you to focus on breathing. But after you get the hang of it and if you want to spend long periods of time on the balls, watching TV is just fine.) You can wear whatever clothing you like, but it should be loose fitting and comfortable.

Next, read Chapter Two on breathing. Breathing is a crucial part of enabling your muscles to release their tension. You may think you are breathing even now as you read this, but most people I know hold their breath almost as much as they actually breathe.

After you have read Chapter Two and have become familiar with how you breathe, choose a body part you'd like to start working on and turn to the chapter on it. Each chapter includes basic positions and variations; please get comfortable with the former before moving on to the latter. In fact, I suggest that you try no more than one position per day to fully experience the process. If you jump from one body part to the next on the same day, you will miss out on many of the benefits of these exercises.

This is difficult for a lot of people to do because they believe the quicker they move on to the next position, the quicker they will see results. Try to be patient. Your body loves to unwork those tight muscles and needs time to do so.

What will unworking your muscles feel like? Imagine wadding a piece of Saran Wrap into a tight ball and leaving it on your kitchen counter. In an hour, the Saran Wrap will relax and you won't have a tight ball anymore. Your muscles will undergo a similar process. They start out tight, tense, and stiff, but as you let your body relax into the balls, your muscles will begin to loosen. Your spine can then begin to realign itself, and pinched nerves can begin to relax. Move through the ball therapy exercises slowly to ensure you get the benefits of each one.

To master each position, follow the instructions for placing the balls under whichever body part you've chosen and let yourself sink into the balls. This is very different from exercises that most people are familiar with. It's the laziest bodywork in the world. I say that because you are going to get more results by working less. That's not a gimmick. Our habit is to push and muscle our body into position, even if it feels uncomfortable or painful. You need to learn how to let go of the tension built up in your muscles. Your goal is to let your weight release and be absorbed by the balls. You will simply breathe and let your muscles unwind. You aren't really going to "do" much else. And that is something many of my students find the most

Don't fix it; feel it. Feeling it is enough. Your body will do the rest.

challenging part of my program—the notion of "un-doing." They are doers—used to achieving goals, fixing problems, being in control—they have a hard time believing that anything can be accomplished by doing nothing at all. It doesn't feel right to them. Well, no more. Your new motto should be: No Pain, Much Gain.

Let me say it again: When you are on the ball, simply give in. Remind yourself to let go, and let gravity and the weight of your body do the work for you.

Please be open-minded. Give yourself a chance to enjoy the feeling of your body.

And take notice of yourself when you come off the ball. Perhaps you don't notice a change immediately. Some of you will and some of you won't. I've had students say to me, "I sleep better at night," or "I'm not as nervous during the day," or "My stomach stopped bothering me," or "I can stand or sit longer periods of time without my back aching." There are many, many changes that may result as you follow this method.

You can do the ball work of any section of the book and feel stress reduction. There is a chain reaction that takes place no matter what body part you've chosen, because all of your parts are ultimately all connected. Thus, even though the pain is in, say, your lower back, you may find great relief from placing the ball under your neck. A bad knee might be helped by hip work. You'll have to tinker to determine which poses suit you best. So find a position that you really love, and spend time with it. If it feels good, then it's good for you, so stay with it. Then you can try other body parts and those will be beneficial, too.

You can enjoy this program in any order you like and you do not have to do every movement in every chapter. Do poses you like; forgo some others. Start with the simplest ones, feel the weight, and allow yourself to breathe. Five to seven minutes in each position is a suggestion for beginners. If you feel able to do 10 or 15 or 20 minutes or more, then it's all the better.

If you experience any kind of discomfort, take the ball away. Pain will make your muscles tense up even more, and with stiff muscles you will not be able to give in to the weight of the ball. Sometimes moving the ball only slightly will relieve discomfort. Even an inch can make for a completely different experience.

Sometimes it's better not to put the ball directly under your problem area. Try a different part of the body, and learn how to do the method there. Unlike most types of exercise, these movements do not isolate one part of the body from the rest. So if you experience the weight of one part of your body giving in, you will eventually feel the domino effect of relief throughout the rest of your body. For example, you might be surprised to find that your tennis elbow is helped by placing the balls under your knees.

Why *Whole Body Moves*?

The Whole Body Moves (which don't involve balls at all) that conclude every chapter should be done each time you finish a session of ball therapy. As you practice them, you will begin to notice how much more fluid your movements are. You may notice that your range of motion is better. You may feel more flexible. Your posture may have improved. Noting these changes in your body, whether you consciously realize it or not, will enable you to gently correct the alignment and tension problems you may be experiencing.

Whole Body Moves are designed to make your body move as an integrated whole. You will probably feel muscles stretching that you've never felt before, especially the hamstrings, those surrounding the hip joints, and those in the back. This is normal and to be expected, so don't be alarmed if the feeling is awkward to you. Try to distinguish between the pain associated with the use of unfamiliar muscles—good pain—and the pain associated with strained muscles—bad pain. If this doesn't make sense to you, think of good pain as similar to the pain associated with an intense massage—it may hurt a little, but it feels good at the same time. This good pain is the kind you have to work through; if you don't continue to move, you won't break your cycle of pain.

Whole Body Moves may resemble stretches to you and, indeed, they will stretch your body. I generally avoid using the word "stretch," because I find people push and push when they stretch, and their muscles shorten as a result, instead of lengthen. As you do the Whole Body Moves, focus on using your weight to pull rather than using your muscles to push. For example, if the Whole Body Move involves you standing up and bending at the hips, hanging your hands toward your feet, you should let the weight of your shoulders and torso pull your hands closer to your feet, rather than engaging your muscles in an attempt to reach for the floor. Whole Body Moves lengthen your muscles, which is what motivates a lot of my students to continue using this program. They discover that their long muscles make them look leaner. As pleased as they are about the potential health benefits of this method, they love their improved shapes even more.

Your posture and the way you move have a big impact on your overall appearance. When you stand straight and move with ease, you look and feel younger. Most people only ever use a small group of muscles, but The Miracle Ball Method will help you "find your parts," as I like to say, and show you how to encourage forgotten muscles to move in new ways. Pay attention to the way you walk throughout the day, and notice how your movements change over time as you practice your ball therapy. As you walk, concentrate on your leg joints, think about your upper back, and lengthen your neck. If you are conscious of the way your body moves, you will be able to change it.

A few final thoughts before you begin:

• As suggested throughout the book, practice your favorite breathing exercise while you are on the ball.

• Conclude each ball therapy session with a Whole Body Move.

• Don't do any move that causes you pain.

• You can use the exercises in any order that feels right to you. Just be sure to read each section carefully to familiarize yourself with the instructions.

• Don't slavishly follow the photos. These are meant as a general guide. Everybody is different, and it's important you don't force your body into positions it isn't ready for.

CHAPTER TWO

How to Breathe

Breathing is an essential component of my method, so I beg you to read this crucial chapter. You may, as I once did, have the idea that breathing is something that comes naturally, that you don't really have to do anything about it. Of course, to some extent that's true. But it is also true that breathing is greatly inhibited by excess muscle tension. Like many people, if you are experiencing other kinds of stress including back pain, you are probably holding your breath. Shallow breathing is very common; correcting your breathing is the first step to pain relief.

First ask yourself: Are you breathing? It may sound like an odd question, but take a moment to answer it. Don't force yourself to breathe; just think about how you are doing it. How would you describe it? Do you breathe with ease? Does it seem to fill your chest and back? Is your exhalation as long as your inhalation? At various times throughout the day, think about whether you are holding your breath. Most of us do.

Just the act of rushing from place to place makes us begin to hold our breath during the day. You don't even have to be doing something taxing. It could be that you have a lot of fun things planned for the day: the kids' piano recital, people over for dinner, a movie. Most of us try to pack a lot into one day. The physical reaction to just the sheer quantity of tasks we have to fulfill each day is to breathe with our upper chests. The diaphragm, which is a muscle responsible for pulling air deeper into the lungs, gets weak and flabby, like any other underutilized muscle. As a result, muscles throughout the body do not receive the oxygen they need in order to remain flexible and unstressed. This is especially true of neck and shoulder pain, which can often be lessened with breath work alone.

Don't concentrate on forcing yourself to breathe all day. The goal in this chapter is to get you breathing naturally from your diaphragm. Your diaphragm is a muscle that sits flat across your body just below your lungs. (I think of it as the skin of a drum, stretching around your ribcage.) A stronger diaphragm will have an easier time pulling air into your lungs and will prevent you from holding your breath. That, in concert with giving in to the weight of your body, will enable you to inhale and exhale fully— maybe for the first time in many years. After some practice, you will notice that breathing properly is easier, and that after a while it has become second nature to you. Your muscles will be able to relax, which in turn will allow you to breathe even more freely. This is how you begin to reverse your cycle of pain.

You can do these exercises anywhere. If the exercises seem too strange or too time-consuming, try them for just five minutes. Then try it again for five minutes the next day. You may be surprised to find how much more energy you have and how much it reduces your anxiety. As you become more comfortable with the exercises, gradually increase the time you spend practicing them.

Fifteen to 20 minutes a day is ideal, but don't feel you have to focus only on breathing. Do breath work along with the Seated Body Hang Over (page 133) or while lying on the ball—just be sure to include it in your ball practice.

Do You Fully Exhale?

Most people inhale much more fully than they exhale, which can elevate the amount of oxygen in the body. Even just a little extra oxygen can explain episodes of dizziness, blurry vision, or light-headedness (which I know from personal experience). This mild state of hyperventilation is much more common than most people realize. Exhaling fully was the solution that worked for me. If you do experience any of these symptoms, however, please check them out with your doctor to rule out anything more serious.

Exercise One

- **The "S" sound**
- **relieves anxiety, tense muscles, and fatigue**

1 Make an "S" sound as you exhale. This sound is one of the ways to strengthen your diaphragm by making you more aware of your exhalation.

Make the sound of an "S" during the entire exhalation. SSSSSSSSSSSSSSSSSSSSSS

Try to make that "S" sound as loud and long as you can.

2 After you run out of air, stop making the sound and notice the difference in your breathing. You should be starting to breathe more deeply and to feel the breath being pulled lower into your lungs. You might feel reactions to the breathing in places that are your tightest areas. Some people begin yawning; others' eyes tear, others feel nothing. It doesn't matter if you feel nothing; the exercise is still helping you breathe properly, and eventually you will notice improvement. Return to the way you normally breathe. Does it feel any different? Looser? Deeper, maybe? Take

note of the changes, then make the "S" sound again.

> **Think "let it happen" while you breathe, not "force it deeper."**

3 Repeat the "S" sound for 5 to 7 minutes a day if you're a beginner. When you feel able to, there is nothing wrong with making the "S" sound for 10, 15, or 20 minutes at a time. But be aware that 5 minutes of observing your reactions following the exercise and allowing your

Yawning

Yawning is a common reaction to making the "S" sound. Do not resist yawning. It is an excellent physical reaction. When you yawn, your lungs fill with air and your abdominal muscles flex, causing the diaphragm to spasm and pull more air into your lungs. It's a corrective measure that your body is doing in order to bring in the oxygen it needs. It probably means that you do hold your breath often, and your body is doing a wonderful thing by taking care of you.

breathing to change will do more for you than 20 minutes of mindless, distracted "S" sounds.

Make the "S" sound as loudly and for as long as you can. Right before the end of the exhalation, stop and notice how you feel.

Be more of an observer than a director. Your goal is to respond to your body's changes, not tell it what to do.

- **Open Mouth Breathing**
- **relieves tight facial muscles and neck and shoulder tension**

1 Hold your hand a few inches in front of your mouth. Open your mouth and exhale for as long as you can, making a hushed "haaa" sound as if you were trying to fog up a cold window. Feel the weight of your jaw as you exhale. Just like any other area of your body, your jaw has weight. Try to become aware of that weight when you open your mouth, but don't force it.

2 At the end of the exhalation, slowly bring your lips together (don't clench your teeth) and notice if there is any change in your breathing. You may have the same reactions as you did during the "S" exercise (see page 65).

3 Repeat this breath work for 5 to 7 minutes. Do you feel your breath filling the back and sides of the rib cage, abdominal area, chest, or shoulders? You may notice some discomfort in your back muscles or feel the need to move your body. This is because the oxygen is beginning to move muscles that have been clenched; until it gets into those areas fully, you may feel a need to relieve that discomfort by stretching—like you do when you wake up in the morning.

Exercise Three

Some common reactions to making the "S" sound and doing open-mouth breathing, as mentioned, are eye tearing, feeling the need to stretch, runny nose, yawning, etc. (If you have a strong urge to stretch, do any one of the Whole Body Moves throughout the book.) One less common reaction is light-headedness. Although the feeling is uncomfortable, it is a positive sign. As a result of your expelling more breath, you are now taking in more oxygen—probably much more than you are used to. Your muscles need to absorb that oxygen. This exercise helps redirect the oxygen to your muscles, thus alleviating your light-headedness.

1 Make fists with both hands and bring them into your chest.

2 Straighten your arms, keeping your fists closed.

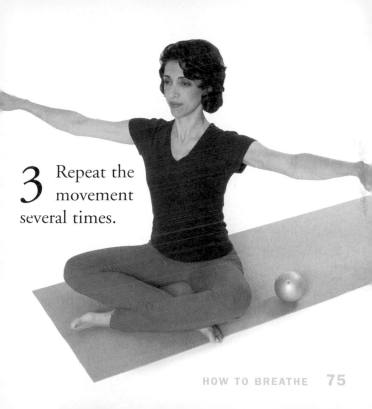

3 Repeat the movement several times.

Exercise Four

- **Tapping**
- **promotes energy restoration; relieves neck and shoulder tension**

1 Cup your hand and tap your upper rib cage, near your collarbone. Instead of focusing on pushing down, focus on pulling away from the skin. Tap in a circular motion and with the same frequency as you use to applaud. Do this for 15 seconds.

2 Lower your hand and notice any changes. Your upper chest may feel warmer or the muscle tension might be lessened. Bring your attention to the feeling in this area. Increased breath leads to awareness of feeling, which leads to more freedom of movement.

3 Repeat the exercise for 5 to 7 minutes, tapping for 15 seconds and then resting for 15 seconds.

In addition to the upper chest above the breast, I like to tap on my shoulder above the clavicle (collarbone) and on the side of my rib cage. All three locations are ideal because tapping there helps loosen the muscles that may be preventing your lungs from fully expanding as you breathe.

At first, many people have a hard time believing that tapping works to relieve muscle tension, but the proof is in the tapping. Try tapping just one side of your body—your left shoulder, for instance. After five minutes of tapping, move your left arm as though you are brushing your hair. Then repeat the motion using your right arm. Most people notice that their left shoulder is much more flexible than the right shoulder.

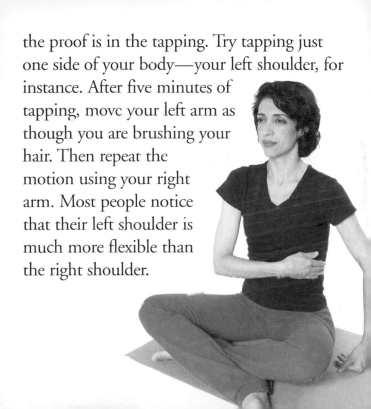

PART TWO

On the Basi

CHAPTER THREE

Back on the Ball

B ack pain is usually caused by one of three things: misalignment of the body, stress, or an injury. Any one or all three of these conditions can put stress on many systems in your body, activating the cycle of pain. When you experience pain, you tend to hold your breath. When you hold your breath, your muscles tighten more, causing more pain and inhibiting your body's natural ability to align itself.

Some people get caught up in their diagnoses. "If I only knew what's wrong, I'd be able to fix it." Whatever your diagnosis, whether you agree with it or whether you don't have one at all, the solution is the same. If you relieve the muscle tension and improve the flexibility of your muscles, you will feel better, no matter what the underlying cause of the pain.

When people are in pain, their instinct is to not move, lest they worsen the pain or injury. Many suppose that they cannot be healed by anyone but a chiropractor, surgeon, or other medical professional. It is your body's own alignment system, in fact, that will relieve your pain. And the way to engage that system is to move *differently*, not to lie still. Of course, there is nothing wrong with going to your doctor, but don't get caught up in the search for a "cure." Back pain is not a disease. It is a result of the condition of your whole body and how you have been caring for it (or ignoring it). Even sciatic pain, which is caused by one of your spinal disks pressing on the sciatic nerve, benefits from reducing muscle tension because pressure on the nerve is aggravated by the increased gripping of tight muscles.

Benefits of Doing Back on the Ball

Back on the Ball is excellent for lengthening the lower spine, for realigning the lumbar vertebrae, and for loosening the leg joints—all of which work to relieve backaches. It is also wonderful for your breathing, keeps the alignment of your legs in balance, and helps your lower abdominal muscles flatten. All of the Back on the Ball movements are great for stress reduction. Pregnant women may find that they help prenatal stomach discomfort. And gardeners and golfers may experience relief from the strains of their pursuits.

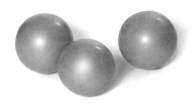

Exercise One

- **Finding Your Hip Joints**
- **relieves stiff lower back muscles and hip joints**

Healing back pain begins with awareness of feeling. Most people don't have feeling in key parts of their body because of excess muscle tension. Let's make sure you are clear on exactly where your hip joints are and how they feel. Tight hip joints, you may be surprised to learn, can be the cause of some kinds of back pain.

When these hip joints are tight, they can pull on your back, causing strain and sometimes knocking it out of alignment.

1 Lie down on the floor with your legs outstretched.

Notice the spaces under your back. Could you drive a truck through the arch

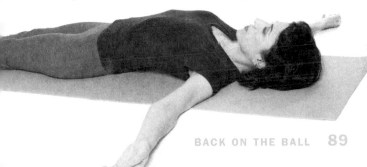

Don't fix it; just feel it.

under your lower back or is most of your
back comfortably resting? Don't try to fix
anything; just feel it.

2 Bend your knees and rest your feet
on the floor.

Does your back flatten
out? See how naturally
it happened when you
bent your knees. As you start to feel where

your hip joints are positioned and realize how they influence your back muscles, your back will begin to rest easier without your knees being bent. When you stand, you will start to transfer your weight away from your back and onto your legs, where it belongs.

3 Repeat extending and bending your knees—very slowly—a few times.

You may start to notice that your back is pulled off the floor when your legs are extended, or outstretched, because of your hip joint. The muscles surrounding the joint where your thigh meets your pelvis are usually very tight. Once you loosen those up, you will experience tremendous relief in your entire back.

- **Back on the Ball**
- **relieves lower backache; promotes relaxation**

This exercise calls for you to put just one ball under your back. If you feel wobbly or unstable this way, please feel free to use two balls. Place one on either side of your tailbone for maximum support.

You may notice some small movements in your body as you rest on the ball. This is very common. Do not resist by clenching your muscles in an effort to remain still. These movements mean that your body's natural alignment system is beginning to work. Your body is trying to find its balance. If you feel like the movements become so big that you are going to fall off the ball, it means you are holding your breath and have lost the sense of your weight sinking into the ball. Try breathing and feeling the weight of your body. If you can't, come off of the ball and try again from the start.

1 Lie on the floor. Bend your knees and rest your feet flat on the mat.

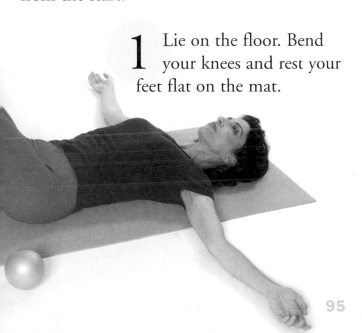

2 Take a ball, roll your pelvis to the side, and place the ball in the middle of the back of your pelvis.

The exact placement of the ball is flexible. You may place it as far down as your tailbone or as far up as the middle of your pelvis. The lower you set it, the easier the exercise will be for you. Do not move the ball up to the top of the pelvis, at your waistline.

That location is usually the tightest, most painful part of a person's back and is too advanced a move to start with. Furthermore, the lower down you place the ball, the more likely you will be able to loosen up your leg joints, which is crucial to this exercise.

3 Roll your pelvis up onto the ball. Feel the weight of your pelvis give in to the ball. Most people

HAMMOCK

VIOLIN BOW

have strong arches in their backs caused by tight, stiff back muscles. They carry their bodies like violin bows. If your back did not rest comfortably on the floor in Exercise One, then you, too, have tight muscles. When you place the ball in this exercise, see if you can get it under your tailbone. This way your spine will hang down from your tailbone like a hammock. The weight of your pelvis will help to lengthen your back muscles as the hammock hangs from rib cage to tailbone. Remember. Don't fix it; just feel it. Let your body do the work.

4 Make the "S" sound.

This is to ensure that you are not holding your breath.

5 One at a time, bring your legs up toward your chest. Give in to the weight of your legs.

Feel the weight of your pelvis give in to gravity. Stay in this position for 2 to 3 minutes. Don't force your knees to go all the way to your chest; let them go as close as they comfortably can. Over time

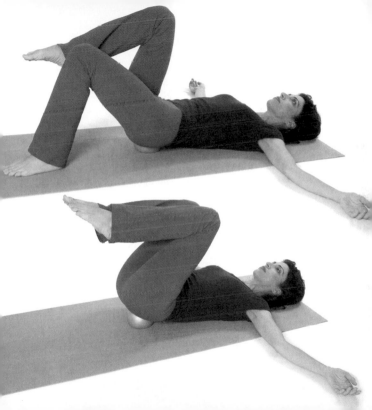

your leg joints will become more flexible and you will be able to get your legs closer to your chest.

Make sure you are not bringing your knees so far up that your pelvis is no longer releasing its weight onto the ball. It doesn't matter how far up you can bring your legs.

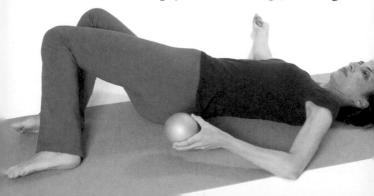

It's important to let the ball absorb your body's weight.

6 Take your feet down one at a time to the bent knee position. Roll your pelvis to the side and quickly take the ball away.

It's important to remove the ball quickly so that you don't tense your muscles again when you lower yourself back to the floor. Let your muscles remain supple and let the weight of your pelvis sink into the floor.

Don't hold your breath. *Breathe.*

7 Rest on your back as you slide your feet out to straighten your knees.

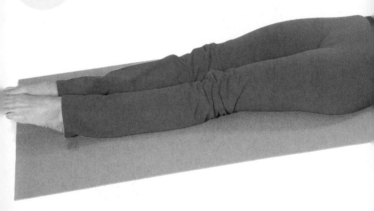

Observe. What is your relationship to the floor? Many people find their lower backs rest closer to the floor, which means that their muscles are more relaxed and have lengthened. Others notice that they are breathing more easily than they were when they first lay down. Maybe you won't notice anything different. That's okay; it will not impede your progress. It can take a while to regain feeling in the body. Eventually you will notice changes.

8 Repeat this exercise 2 to 3 times.

I recommend to my students with back pain that they do this very basic exercise every day, remembering that it is not work. It is unwork—there should be no effort here. The whole process takes about 10 minutes. If you want to do it longer, feel free.

- **Back on the Ball with Inner Thigh Release**
- **loosens lower back muscles; reshapes hips and thighs; helps realign hip joints**

This is an excellent exercise for people who tend to roll their knees in toward one another when they walk and for people with foot pain.

1 Do the basic movement for Back on the Ball (page 93) and bring your legs up to your chest.

2 Slowly let your thighs move apart, keeping your pelvis anchored on the ball.

Let your thighs move as far apart as they comfortably can. Do not force them wide. Rest in this position as long as you can for up to 2 minutes. Most of us have very tight inner thigh muscles. It may appear that the muscle is flabby, and it's true—the muscle on the surface, that is. But the muscle that is wrapped around the joint is exceedingly tight and stiff. This example of imbalance in tone not only looks bad but, worse, could lead to knee and foot injuries. It is essential to relax these muscles.

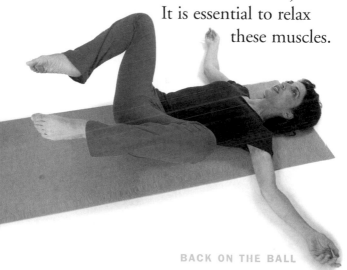

3 Slowly bring your thighs back to the starting position. Feel the weight of your legs and go very slowly.

Place your hands on the outside of your buttocks as you bring your legs together so you can feel the muscles on

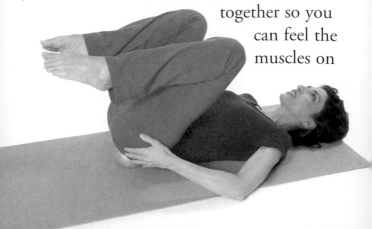

the sides of your thighs working. Let your knees follow your thighs, rather than leading with your knees as many people do.

4 Repeat the spreading and closing of your thighs 3 times.

Each time make sure to feel the weight of your legs.

Are you feeling this in other parts of your body? Remember to make the "S" sound as you breathe.

5 One at a time, return your feet to the floor with your knees bent, as in the basic Back on the Ball exercise (page 103). Roll your pelvis to the side and quickly take the ball away.

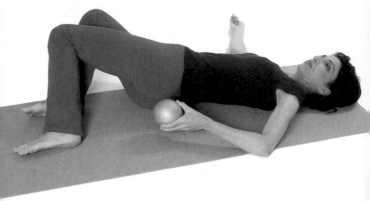

- **Back on the Ball with Quadricep Stretch**
- **slims the thighs; stretches abdomen; strengthens hips**

1 Do the basic movement for Back on the Ball (page 93) to bring your knees up to your chest.

2 Clasp your fingers over your right knee.

Let the weight of your hands draw your knee closer to your shoulder. Try not to stiffen your shoulders.

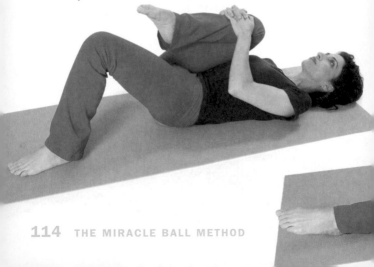

3 Gently place your left foot on the floor and slide it away from your pelvis.

Straighten your knee joint as much as you comfortably can. Don't force it and don't hyperextend it. Rest in this position for 1 minute.

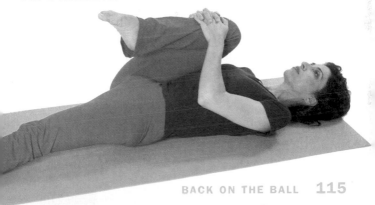

4 Flex and extend both of your ankles and heels.

Flex for 10 to 15 seconds, then point the toes for 10 to 15 seconds.

5 Place your right foot on the floor and slide it forward, and rest with both legs stretched out.

For some people this is one of the best poses for releasing the back. If you find it comfortable, feel free to stay in the position as long as you like, doing one of your favorite breathing exercises. Remember that feeling good is your body's way of telling you that a pose is beneficial to it.

6 Repeat the exercise with your left leg.

This time grasp your left knee and slide your right foot away from your pelvis. Flex and point your feet, then straighten your left leg on the floor and rest.

7 Do 3 repetitions, alternating each side.

**Remember to breathe. Make the
"S" sound.**

8 Return both feet to the floor with your
knees bent, roll your pelvis to the side,
and quickly remove the ball.

Exercise Five

- **Back on the Ball with Legs up the Wall**
- **relieves stiff hamstrings; releases lower back and hips**

1 Do the basic movement for Back on the Ball (page 93) and bring your legs, bent at the knees, to your chest.

2 Pretend your feet are resting flat against a wall and slide them straight up this imaginary wall.

Try to avoid stiffening your legs. Let the weight of your pelvis be your anchor. Do not let your feet drift and end up above your face. They should be directly over your hip joints. If you have a problem imagining the wall, feel free to use a real wall. Slide your feet up the real wall and let them rest on it.

3 Leave your legs against the wall for up to 1 minute.

4 Bring your knees down so that they are bent against your chest. Feel their weight.

5 Repeat 3 times.

6 Return your feet to the floor with your knees bent, roll your pelvis to the side, and quickly remove the ball.

Exercise Six

- **Back on the Ball with Inner Thigh Rotation**
- **engages weak inner thigh muscles;
  relieves tight hip joints**

1 Do the basic movement for Back on the Ball (page 93) and bring your legs, bent at the knees, to your chest.

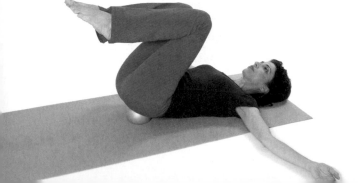

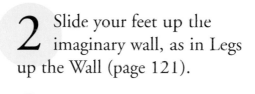

2 Slide your feet up the imaginary wall, as in Legs up the Wall (page 121).

3 Take the second ball and put it between your upper thighs.

Remember to keep breathing.

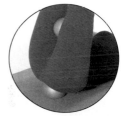

Locate the inner thigh muscles that are closest to the ball. The ball is there to create feeling and to connect your brain to unfamiliar or underused parts of your body. The inner thigh muscles are essential for keeping us upright and are directly connected to our lower back muscles.

4 Very slowly rotate your thighs around the ball for 1 minute.

Gently turn your thighs as far as is comfortable, first inward toward one another, and then outward. Don't let your knees make the movement happen, let the rotation come from the hip joint. Your knees are overused and you will get better results if you use your hip, even if you make a smaller rotation with it.

Initiate movement from the part of your body that is in contact with the ball.

5 Slowly bend your knees toward your chest and let your thighs open. (The ball will fall out.) Rest there for 1 minute.

If you need to, place your feet on the floor and stretch out your legs. Notice your breathing. Let a chain reaction move through your body, as one relaxed body part encourages others to loosen. Then remove the ball.

6 Repeat these steps 3 times.

7 Return your feet to the floor, and with your knees bent, roll your pelvis to the side and quickly remove the ball.

- **Back on the Ball with Hamstring Stretch**
- improves leg circulation; relieves back pain

1 Do the basic movement for Back on the Ball (page 93) and bring your legs, bent at the knees, to your chest.

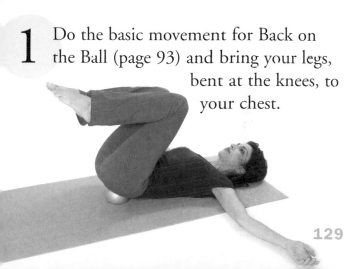

2 Slide your feet up the imaginary wall, as in Legs up the Wall (page 121).

3 With your legs together, shift your weight gently to your left side and lean into the left hip.

Rest there for 10 to 15 seconds, feeling the stretch down the back of that hip.

This is a very subtle movement for more mobility in the lower back; you don't need to make large movements. Small movements will help the tension in your lower back more than ambitious ones will.

4 Shift your weight gently to your right side and lean into the right hip.

Rest there for 10 to 15 seconds, feeling the stretch down the back of that hip.

5 Repeat 3 times on each side.

Unlike most types of exercise, you don't need to do every ball position in order to benefit. It's better to do one of them really well than to try six or eight while you're clenching your muscles and holding your breath.

6 Return your feet to the floor with your knees bent, roll your pelvis to the side, and quickly remove the ball.

Whole Body Move

- **Seated Body Hang Over**
- **improves breathing and posture; increases flexibility; reduces back pain**

1 Sit on a bench or cross-legged on the floor.

2 Roll your body forward over your legs.

Start with the top of your head and neck and let them bend forward. When your torso is hanging over your legs, stay in that position just long enough to notice if you've started to hold your breath. Breath holding is very common; as soon as most of us begin to move, we stop breathing. This makes it harder to feel the weight of the movement. If you find yourself holding your breath when you hang over, exhale. Hum a tune, or give yourself some other way of making an exhalation happen, and then you won't be able to hold your breath. Then come back up. That could take perhaps 30 seconds. Do this about 3 times after you finish Back on the Ball exercises.

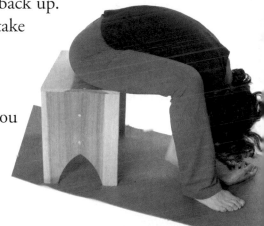

3 Sit up and let your body realign itself.

Let your body respond to feeling its weight and to your deeper breathing. Maybe you notice your chest muscles are looser; maybe you are more comfortably balanced on your stool. You should be more comfortable than before you started. And you should move more naturally than before you started, thanks to the oxygen that is circulating to your muscles more freely.

As your body realigns, consider this. You have three major weights in your body: your pelvis, your rib cage, and your head. When you uncurl your body and return to sitting, notice where these three weights are. Ideally they should be stacked neatly on top of one another like children's building blocks. If they are out of alignment, then you have not yet perfected your balance. Good posture comes more from balance than from forcing body parts into position.

CHAPTER FOUR

Hips and Legs
on the Ball

Your hip—where your thigh meets your pelvis—may be your most important joint. It is the foundation of movement of the entire body. If your hip joints are moving freely, then they absorb the shock of your actions. If they are tight, the shock is absorbed by other areas less able to cope with it, like your back, knees, and neck. When these other areas have to compensate for work that your tight hip joints can't do, the result is stiffness and, often, pain. Unfortunately, most of us have very tight hip joints and tightness in the surrounding leg muscles (especially the hamstrings) that pull at our back and knees, in many cases causing pain. These exercises will relieve back pain, especially sciatic pain, pressure on heel spurs, foot aches, and knee instability.

Exercise One

- **Hips on Two Balls**
- **relieves sciatic pain and hip discomfort**

This movement is a favorite of mine; it is incredibly comfortable and soothing. It is utterly easy to do—it's just resting on two balls placed under the back of the pelvis—and I do it often (sometimes for hours) while I listen to music, watch TV, talk to my family.

Type A readers may resist this one. All you will do is lie on the floor, letting the balls absorb the body's weight. It seems counterintuitive that something so seemingly passive can yield results, but it does work. Just breathe and sink into the balls. No Pain; Much Gain.

1 Lie down on the floor, bend your knees, rest your feet on the floor. Take a ball in each hand.

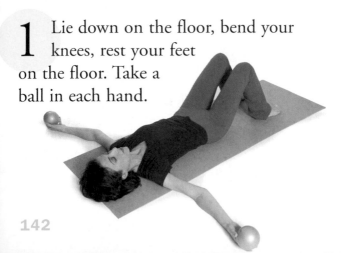

2 Roll your pelvis to one side. Place one ball under the raised side of the pelvis and roll up onto that ball.

The fleshiest part of your buttocks is where the hip joint is located. That is usually the most comfortable place to put the ball.

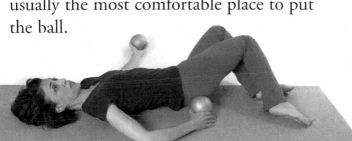

3 Raise the other side of your pelvis and place the other ball under it.

4 Let your body's weight sink into the balls.

Adjust the balls if they feel uneven, being aware that it may be your body that is uneven. If there is a spot that hurts, don't rest on that spot.

5 Rest on the balls for 2 to 3 minutes.

6 Take the balls away: roll your pelvis to one side and remove the free ball. Roll to the other side and remove that ball.

Remember your body formula:
Weight + Breathing = Release of Tension.

7 Extend your legs. Rest for 1 minute without the balls.

If you want to flex your ankles, go right ahead. Then lie still in a neutral position to compare how your whole body rests on the floor to the way it did when you first lay down.

8 Put the balls in a slightly different place under your pelvis; a little lower down or a little farther apart.

9 Rest on the balls again with your legs outstretched for 2 to 3 minutes.

Take notice if you feel any small movements while you are on the balls. You don't have to fix your body; just feel your body and it will fix itself. Observation is powerful, so take notice of your body.

10 Remove the balls as in step 6.

11 Rest for 1 to 2 minutes with your legs extended.

Exercise Two

- **Hips and Thighs Moving Down Two Balls (with rotation)**
- **relieves hip and knee pain; realigns hip joints**

1 Lie down on the floor, bend your knees, and rest your feet flat on the floor. Take a ball in each hand.

2 Roll your pelvis to one side. Place one ball under the raised side of the pelvis and roll up onto that ball.

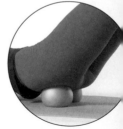

The fleshiest part of your buttocks is where the hip joint is located. That is usually the most comfortable place to put the ball.

3 Raise the other side of your pelvis and place the other ball under it.

4 Let your weight sink into the balls and rest here for several minutes or longer.

5 Slowly extend your legs one after the other, sliding your feet along the floor just as you did in Hips on Two Balls, page 146.

Rest with your legs outstretched for 2 to 3 minutes.

Let your weight sink into the balls. Make the "S" sound to ensure that you are not holding your breath.

6 Tip your weight to one side and push the ball on the opposite side down to the middle of your thigh. Repeat on the other side.

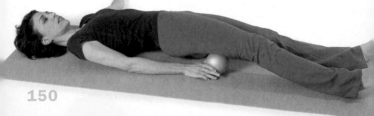

Let the weight of your legs sink into the balls. Try to avoid letting your knees roll in toward one another. If you find they are slumping inward, try adjusting the balls to encourage your knees to roll slightly outward instead.

7 Slowly roll your thighs toward each other and then let them release back to neutral.

This is a very subtle movement. Your goal is simply to release some of the tension in your hips, which may be responsible for knee and hip problems. It should feel like a nice massage. Let the movement start with your hip joints, not your knees. Do 2 or 3 slow rolls.

8 Remove the balls and rest on the floor.

Are you resting closer to the floor? Are you breathing easier? Most people find that they are. If you like, at this point you may go back on the balls, placing one under each of your hip joints. Then, instead of stretching your legs out straight, bend your knees and bring your thighs up to your chest. Do your hips feel more limber? Rest here, if you like, letting your weight sink into the balls and remembering to breathe.

Exercise Three

- **Knee on the Ball**
- **relieves achy knees and sciatic pain; promotes relaxation**

1 Lie down on the floor, take the ball that's nearest you, and place it under one knee.

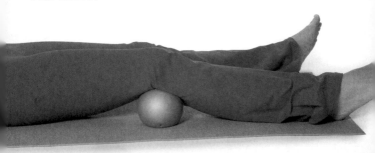

If one side gives you trouble, start with that side. Avoid stiffening your leg when you have your knee on the ball. Let your hip joint rotate if that is what it is inclined to do.

2 Let your knee roll outward from center, keeping it on the ball. This is your starting point.

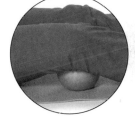

3 Rest on the ball 2 to 3 minutes and then slowly rotate the knee inward until your legs are parallel again.

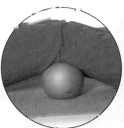

Remember, always adjust the ball to your body; never adjust your body to the ball. If you need to move the ball in order for it to support the part of the body that's resting on it, move the ball. Don't hold your body stiff to try to balance on the ball—your goal is to have this ball completely support the part of the body that's resting on it. That part of the body has to stop working in order to let go. Once that part stops exerting effort, you can feel the weight of that part.

4 Very slowly, release the knee to a neutral position.

As you let go, notice any changes. Maybe your knee is more at ease. Maybe it turns out more easily. You may even notice a difference in your hip or ankle.

5 Take your knee off the ball and rest your leg on the floor.

Try to sense if this side of your body feels different from before.

6 Repeat the exercise with the other knee.

Exercise Four

- **Foot on the Ball**
- **relieves foot pain and stiff leg joints; strengthens ankles**

1 After you do Knee on the Ball (page 154) stay on the floor with the ball under one knee.

You may bend your other leg with your foot flat on the floor (easier), or keep it stretched out straight (more challenging).

2 Bend your knee and raise your leg just enough to rest the bottom of your foot on the ball.

Your knee should form about a 90-degree angle.

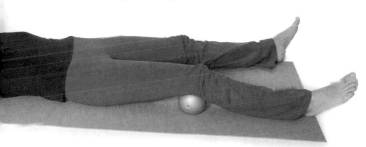

3 Gently move your foot forward and back over the ball for 2 to 3 minutes.

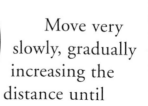

Move very slowly, gradually increasing the distance until

you're rolling the ball all the way from your heel to your toes. Remember to let your ankle bend.

4 Let your leg straighten, rolling the ball close to or directly beneath your ankle.

Rest here for several minutes. Do your breathing work.

5 Raise your knee again, rolling the ball under your heel until your foot rests on the ball. Move your foot back and forth again for 2 to 3 minutes.

Feel what happens to other parts of your body. Do you feel it in your back?

6 Repeat this movement 3 times. Take your leg off the ball and rest it, extended, on the floor.

7 Repeat the same movements with the other leg.

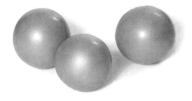

- **Standing Body Hang Over**
- relieves tight back muscles and hamstrings; promotes flexibility; reshapes entire body

This movement is designed to lengthen the muscles from the back of your heels all the way to the back of your neck. A couple of quick hints before we start: (1) Don't stay hung over too long. If you are very stiff, you will feel sharp pulling in the back of your neck and in your hamstrings. Eventually, when you can truly bend at the top of your thigh at your hip joint and release your pelvis over your thighs, you will get relief through your whole back and you will be able to stay bent over longer. (2) Focus on trying to bend at the hip. Most people bend with the exact areas that hurt them, such as the lower back, rather than the hip joint. You need to let your hip act as a hinge and let your legs support you.

A full-length mirror is perfect for use in this exercise. Start by just doing a typical bend over, as if you are going to touch your toes, but don't force anything. Look sideways in the mirror. Many people will find that their buttocks, their sit bones (the pointy bones at the base of the pelvis), and their pelvis are several inches behind their heels. In other words, if you drew a line from the back of their heels to their butt, it would be diagonal, not straight. Usually people also bend their knees, because they don't want to feel that hamstring stretch. Try to straighten your legs (but don't lock your knees) and align your pelvis with your feet as best you can. As you do that, you will feel many body parts stretching, especially your hamstrings.

1 Stand with your feet a little wider than hip-distance apart.

This is the easiest way to start. When you become more flexible, you may move your feet closer together so they are aligned with your hips.

2 Roll your head and body toward your toes, letting your arms hang.

Start from the top of your head and let its weight lead your torso downward. Vertebra by vertebra, let your body give in to gravity. Exhale, make an "S" sound, hum a tune, or whatever you prefer to prevent holding your breath.

Don't try to imitate the photos in this book exactly if it feels uncomfortable. No two bodies are exactly alike and you should not force yourself into any position.

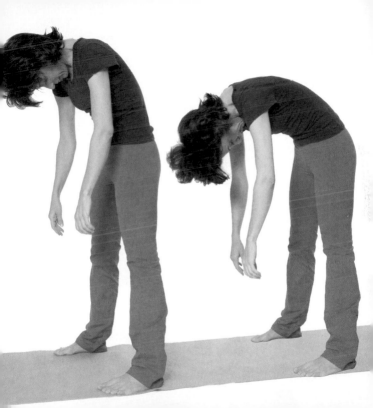

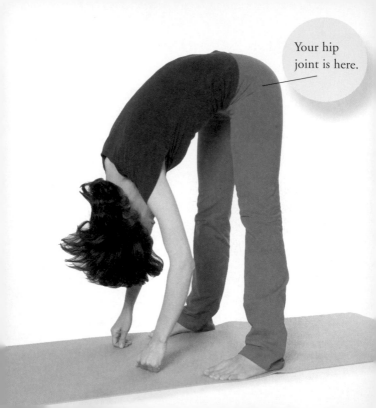

Your hip joint is here.

3 Bend forward from your hips as low as you comfortably can without bending your knees, but without locking them as well.

Notice that your hip joint is a hinge and your pelvis is supporting most of your weight. (You may not feel this at first, depending on how flexible you are.) Stay there. Breathe. Give in to gravity and let go of the muscles in the upper portion of your body, including your neck and your shoulders. Notice that your feet are a firm support here and that your quadriceps and abdominal muscles are engaged.

4 Roll back up, vertebra by vertebra.

5 Repeat 2 times.

Do this 3 times a day. Eventually you will be able to hang over longer and longer as your hamstrings stretch out and you remember how to use your hip joint. Place your hands on your hip joints if you need a reminder of where the motion for this hang should originate.

CHAPTER FIVE

Calves on a Stool

Your pelvis is perfectly aligned with your spine when you are lying on the floor with your calves resting on a flat surface that is about knee height. Most of my students adore this position. Even without the balls it takes the pressure off your lower back, and it makes you realize the importance of loosening those stiff hip joints. It is also an ideal position in which to breathe fully, because your torso is spread out and your diaphragm has room to expand.

Use Calves on a Stool for work with a sore back, knee and hip pain, and abdominal reshaping. Calves on a Stool with Two Balls and Legwork (exercise two) is particularly good for relieving menstrual cramps, stomachaches, and indigestion. Many students who are recovering from childbirth find that this is one of the best positions to gently encourage the abdominal muscles to flatten back into shape.

Exercise One

- **Calves on a Stool**
- **relieves lower back pain (especially during pregnancy); strengthens abdominal muscles**

This exercise is perfect when you need immediate relief from back pain. Use a surface that is 14 to 16 inches high, such as a stool, ottoman, bench, coffee table, or even a crate. (Fourteen to 16 inches is an estimate. What's important is that your feet are not higher than your knees and your calves are roughly parallel to the floor.) You won't need the balls. The position is incredibly relaxing. It puts your pelvis into perfect alignment with the rest of your body and takes all the pressure off of your back muscles. This is because your legs—which are probably tight in the joints and throwing your back out of kilter—are completely supported by the stool. It is also a position that makes breathing easier, as your diaphragm is no longer hindered by the muscle tension in your lower back. Important: Many people use more effort than they need to raise their pelvis. Don't use more effort than is required.

1 Lie on the floor and rest your calves on the stool, so that your knees and feet are parallel to the floor. Important: Your feet must not be higher than your knees.

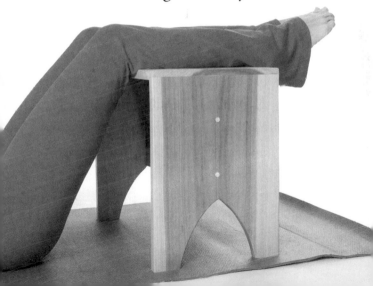

2 With your calves still on the stool, curl the lower half of your pelvis upward, then release it to feel its weight.

Do not lift your pelvis as though to exercise your muscles; curl your pelvis as though you are trying to bring it to touch your nose. You should be curling the pelvis to feel the weight of it when you lower it. It is the lowering in this exercise that is important.

Are you still breathing? Please do; this is a good time to make the "S" or "Haaa" sound. Remember: Weight + Breathing = Release of Muscle Tension

3 Gradually lower your pelvis to the floor.

Don't suddenly drop your pelvis. Feel the weight as you let it down. Take note of the changes. Is more of your back resting on the floor? Do you lean into one hip more than the other? The more you notice, the more you will be able to direct your body to release the muscle tension that may be creating imbalances.

4 Do this for 10 to 15 minutes a day, remembering to breathe.

Exercise Two

- **Calves on a Stool with Two Balls and Legwork**
- **relieves menstrual cramps, hip discomfort and stiffness; aligns hips and legs; reduces stress (a great position for stress reduction)**

1 Move into position for Calves on a Stool (page 175) and insert two balls under your back.

Roll one hip to the side and place a ball under the raised side. Get onto that ball completely as you place the other ball under your other side.

You can always move the balls lower beneath your spine or move them up a few inches. Their location isn't important. What matters is that the position be comfortable and that you be able to feel that the balls are absorbing your weight. The goal here is to unwork the tension in your muscles so that your circulation will improve and you will breathe fully.

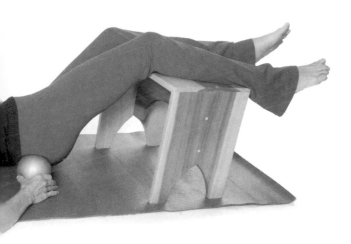

2 With your calves still on the stool, curl the lower half of your pelvis upward, then release it to feel its weight.

Make the "S" sound with your breath and perform 8 to 10 pelvic curls (see pages 178–179). Scan your body to notice whether you are holding your muscles tight in other areas. Focus on giving in to gravity. When you release each curl, notice whether you are sinking farther into the balls. If you are sinking farther, it's a sign that you are successfully reducing your excess muscle tension. If not, on the next repetition, try feeling your weight more and focus on your breathing. Don't take your weight off the balls. You should feel like you are sinking even deeper on to them.

3 With each leg in turn, clasp your fingers on one knee and draw it gently to your chest, then let it

sink back on to the stool. This is great relief for your back.

4 Slide both legs toward you, rest your feet on the near edge of the stool, and let your thighs open.

The weight of your legs stretches out your whole back and your inner thighs. Rest in that position for about 1 minute. (If you cannot do a full minute,

rest in the position as long as you
comfortably can.)

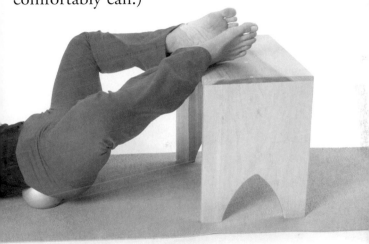

5 Slide your calves back onto the stool, and take the balls away.

Roll your pelvis to one side and quickly remove the free ball; roll your pelvis to the other side and quickly remove the other ball. Do you rest differently on the floor? Do you breathe differently?

6 To come off the stool, roll to the side and rest for a few minutes.

Gently push the stool out of your way before coming up to a sitting position.

- **The Posture Pin**
- **reshapes hips and thighs; realigns entire body; strengthens leg joints and back muscles**

Think of the way young children sit on the floor, their legs casually in front of them, bent at the hips, their backs straight. A great many adults are so far removed from being able to sit on the floor this way, either cross-legged or straight-legged, that they can barely remember how it's done. This Whole Body Move is designed to address that inflexibility. It requires that you sit on a posture pin (or a rolling pin, as it's known in the kitchen), and it enables you to find your hip joint and bend it as you probably haven't done in years.

1 Sit cross-legged on the floor (or as cross-legged as you can).

2 Place a rolling pin behind your hip, hold on to each end with your hands, and lift yourself onto the pin.

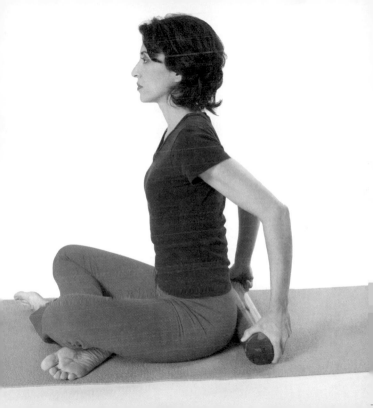

Ideally you are sitting atop your sit bones (the pointy bones at the base of your pelvis). This can be tough for beginners, so some of you are probably hanging just slightly off the back of the pin and others in front of it. If you find that you are very unbalanced, use your hands to stabilize yourself. Remember to breathe.

Breathe, making the "S" sound.

3 Try to balance yourself atop your sit bones.

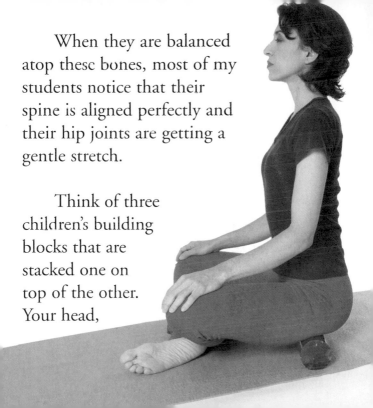

When they are balanced atop these bones, most of my students notice that their spine is aligned perfectly and their hip joints are getting a gentle stretch.

Think of three children's building blocks that are stacked one on top of the other. Your head, rib cage, and pelvis should be stacked similarly. If any one of the blocks is out of alignment, the whole stack is affected.

4 Roll yourself behind your sit bones, so that from the side your body appears to form the letter "C." Then use your pelvis muscles to pull yourself back up onto the tops of the sit bones. Repeat slowly several times.

Notice how your posture is affected in each position and how much deeper into the "C" curve you can sink each time. You are working the most important muscles of your body: those surrounding the hip joints, your lower abs, and hamstrings.

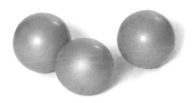

CHAPTER SIX

Head and Neck on the Ball

The muscles supporting the head and neck can, like those supporting the back, be some of the most tense in the body. We tend to hold stress in the neck, which makes the muscles work extra hard to keep the head supported. Head on the Ball exercises will help you get a good night's sleep, as well as prevent headaches. If you include the open mouth breathing work with these movements, you may find relief for the stiff jaw syndrome known as TMJ. Head on the Ball will also reshape the look of your neck and shoulders, and it can release tension far down your back, as well. It's one of my favorite positions because it is so relaxing.

Exercise One

- **Head on the Ball**
- **relieves tension headaches, and neck and shoulder stiffness; promotes stress relief and relaxation**

1 Lie down on the floor with your legs outstretched.

2 Place a ball under your neck.

Use one hand to raise your head and the other to place the ball under your head and neck. The spot most students find comfortable is the place where the base of the skull meets the top of the neck. It feels as if there is a groove there that is just right

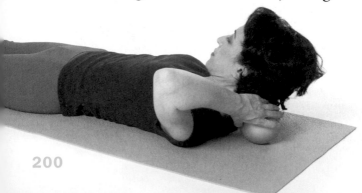

for resting on the ball. Feel the weight of your head as you release tension onto the ball. (Remember: You must be able to feel the weight of your head and neck. Make sure you are not holding tension by pushing your chin into your neck.) Stay in this position for 2 to 3 minutes.

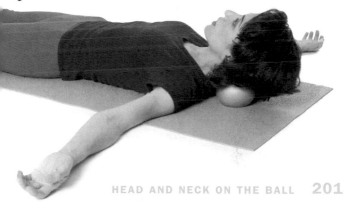

3 Do your open mouth breathing.

4 Take the ball away.

Use one hand to support your head as you quickly remove the ball with the other hand. Then cradle the back of your head in your hand and ease it down to the floor slowly. Let your head rest on the floor and take note of your breathing.

5 Repeat this exercise 3 times, 2 to 3 minutes on the ball, 1 to 2 minutes off.

If you have a tremendous amount of neck tension that you want to release, but you don't feel at ease on the ball just yet, take the ball away more often. This is quite common for beginners, and it's perfectly fine. These exercises are not about staying on the ball; they are about being able to give in to your body's weight when you come off the ball.

Awareness is the key to change.

Exercise Two

- **Head on the Ball with Gentle Neck Turns**
- **lengthens upper back muscles; reshap upper body; relieves stress, eyestrain, and insomnia**

I cannot stress enough how slowly you need to move when you do this exercise. Your movement should be completely imperceptible to someone watching you.

1 Do the basic movement for Head on the Ball (page 199).

2 When you are up on the ball, and you have allowed yourself to rest in the basic position for at least 1 minute, allow

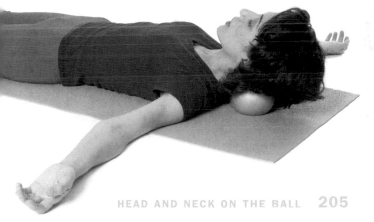

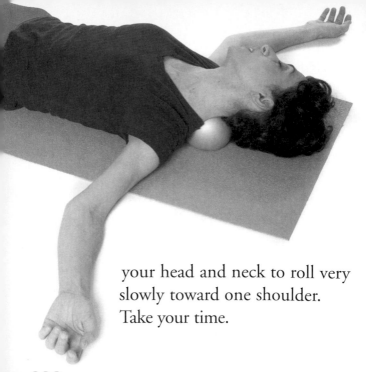

your head and neck to roll very
slowly toward one shoulder.
Take your time.

Let the weight of your head on the ball be your focus. Observe the weight very slowly moving.

Once you have released the weight of your head, it will want to build momentum. Don't allow this to happen. Also, do not feel that you have to make an effort to roll your head over as far as possible. That is not the point of this movement.

If you feel you are going to fall off the ball when you turn your head, don't turn your head as far. Eventually, as you

feel more of the weight of your head, you will also feel more secure on the ball.
Take as much time as you need if it feels good. It is fine to take 5 to 10 minutes to go from one side to the other.

3 Once you've gone as far as you comfortably can toward one shoulder, take your time and come back to center.

Remember to breathe while you do this.

4 Repeat to the other side.

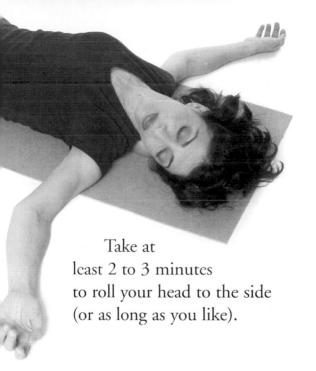

Take at
least 2 to 3 minutes
to roll your head to the side
(or as long as you like).

5 When your head comes back to the starting point, tilt it up and down on the ball in slow motion, as if you were

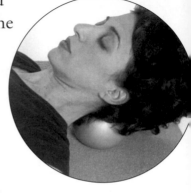

nodding yes to someone. Nod just as slowly as when you moved your head from side to side.

6 Take the ball away.

Use one hand to support your head as you quickly remove the ball with the other hand. Then cradle the back of your head in your hand and ease it slowly down to the floor. Let your head rest on the floor, and take notice of your breathing.

Exercise Three

- **Head on the Ball with Gentle Neck Rolls**
- **relieves tension in face, jaw, and middle back; decreases stress and fatigue**

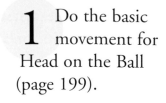

1 Do the basic movement for Head on the Ball (page 199).

2 When you are up on the ball, and you have allowed yourself to rest in the basic position for at least 1 minute, slowly start drawing circles in the air with the tip of your nose.

Imagine that the tip of your nose is a Magic Marker, and very slowly draw small circles to the left (in other words, counter-clockwise) and then to the right (clockwise), 5 to 6 times in each direction.

3 Remember to breathe. A good way to remind yourself to continue breathing is to do open mouth breathing. Make the "S" sound or the "Haaa" sound.

4 Now take the ball and place it slightly lower down the back of your neck.

Notice the different feeling and position of your head. It should tip gently away from your body. Rest for 2 to 3

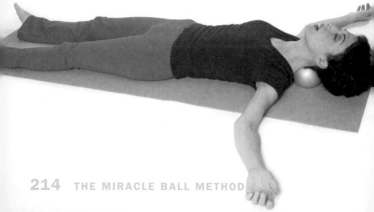

minutes like this, letting your head give in to its weight. Breathe.

5 Push the ball farther down one more time and rest in this position for 2 to 3 minutes.

6 Take the ball away. Use one hand to support your head as you quickly remove the ball with the other hand. Then cradle the back of your head in your hand and ease it to the floor right away. Let your head rest on the floor, and take notice of your breathing.

- **The Ceiling Gaze**
- **lengthens neck and upper back muscles; relieves upper back stiffness; improves posture**

Remember this as you work: The body places the head in the correct position. The head does not place the body into the correct position. Think of your head as a marble bust that rests on a mantel. The mantel holds up the bust; the bust can't hold itself up, nor can it move the mantel into a different position. The mantel provides the base and the strength.

1 Sit on the floor or a hard wooden chair. Face straight ahead.

Notice how your head sits atop your body. Some of you may hold your chin several inches in front of your chest. Or you may rest your head on your rib cage or tilt it to one side.

2 Slowly turn your head and neck to the right, then to the left.

Bring your chin over your shoulder as far as you can without strain. What is happening to your body? Most people feel a stretch in several areas: between the shoulders, in the lower back, even in the hips and thighs.

3 Repeat 3 times.

4 Move your head back to the starting point and take notice of your posture again. Do breathing exercises for 1 minute.

There are only two types of responses when you move a part of your body: stiffening and loosening. Stiffening increases tension and aggravates pain. Loosening allows your body to realign itself and prevents injury.

5 Slowly let go of your chin until it is resting on your chest. Allow your head and neck to follow and hang without letting your shoulders move forward. Stay in position for 5 to 10 seconds. Notice if you feel a stretch between the shoulder blades.

Then slowly raise your head until it's upright.

6 Slowly move your head backward, so that you are looking toward the ceiling.

The ceiling gaze can be one of the most difficult positions, as it is a movement most of us seldom do. To make it easier for you, reach your hands up toward the ceiling and gaze at your hands. Then bend your elbows, clasping your hands behind your head to gently support it. Arch back further, stretching the back of your neck and the uppermost part of your chest.

Finish by returning your arms to your sides and your gaze forward. Do this 3 to 4 times, moving from resting your chin on your chest to lifting your chin in the air.

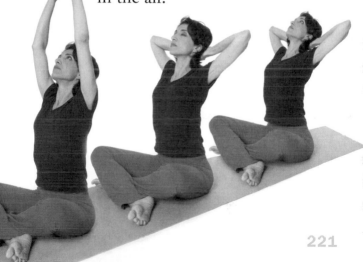

CHAPTER SEVEN

Elbow on the Ball

Elbow exercises? Many of my students with pain in other areas of their body, as well as most of those seeking treatment for anxiety or depression, do not believe that elbow exercises will help them. They figure that the elbow is not close enough to the focus of their problems to do any good. In fact, Elbow on the Ball is one of the best movements they can do. It helps loosen the shoulder joints, neck, and lower back all at once. By enabling you to feel the weight of your arm, it allows your shoulder joints to rotate and loosens the muscles along the spine. This can also provide relief from frozen shoulders, tension headaches, anxiety, and poor posture.

When your elbow is on the ball, do not feel that you have to force your hand to the floor if it doesn't naturally reach it. My hand reaches the floor because my shoulder rotates easily. Never adjust your body to the ball; adjust the ball to your body.

1 Lie down on the floor with your arms outstretched.

Notice how your body rests on the floor. If one

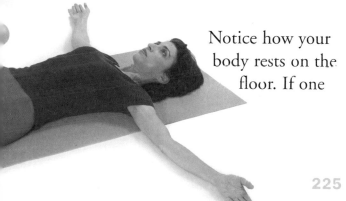

side seems tighter or more painful than the other, work on that side first.

2 Let's say your left side is tighter. Take the ball in your right hand. Make a right angle with your left arm, then place the ball under that elbow joint.

If your right side is tighter, take the ball in your left hand and place it under the crook of the right elbow. Let the weight of your elbow give in to the ball. Try to feel your whole arm and shoulder sinking in to the ball. Stay in position for 2–3 minutes.

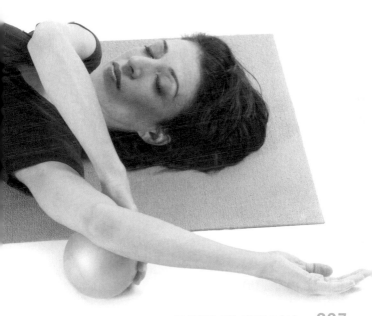

Some people find it difficult to keep the ball under their elbow and it rolls out of place. If this happens to you, move the ball toward your body so it rests under the crease that forms when you bend your arm 90 degrees, rather than on the outside of your elbow. It is easier to give in to the ball in that position without fear of losing it. Let your hand rest as close to the floor as comes naturally. Eventually your shoulders will rotate and your hands will rest on the floor.

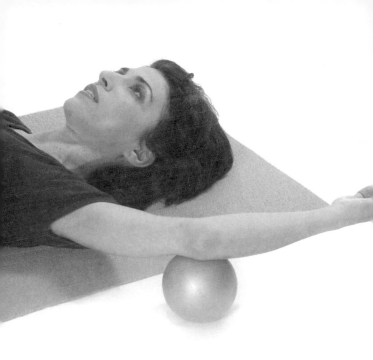

3 Remove the ball.

Give in to the weight of your arm. Are you resting any differently on the floor? Compare the arm and shoulder you just worked with to your other arm and shoulder. As you give in to the weight of your arm, is it easier to take deep, full breaths?

4 Repeat the movement 3 times, 2 to 3 minutes on the ball, 1 to 2 minutes off.

5 Switch sides and repeat with the other elbow.

- **Arm Roll**
- **relieves carpal tunnel syndrome, tight shoulder muscles, mid-back discomfort, and tennis elbow**

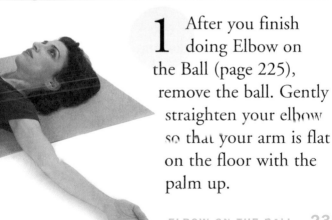

1 After you finish doing Elbow on the Ball (page 225), remove the ball. Gently straighten your elbow so that your arm is flat on the floor with the palm up.

ELBOW ON THE BALL **231**

2 Roll the arm so that the palm is down.

Use your whole arm, starting at the shoulder joint, not just your elbow or just your hand. Remember to feel the weight of your arm. This is easiest to do when the arm is as relaxed as possible. Every time the palm is turned toward the ceiling, let it rest there for a moment while you sense your arm's weight and take notice of your breathing.

3 Roll your arm from palm up to palm down 3 times.

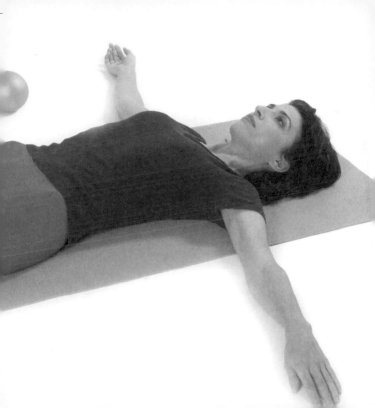

- **Whole Body Twist**
- **slims waist; improves posture; increases energy and breathing; relieves back pain**

This Whole Body Move helps the muscles around your spine become more flexible. Remember as you do it not to force your shoulder to move. Your torso and back should be doing most of the moving in this exercise.

1 Roll onto your left side and rest your right knee on the floor just in front of your left knee.

If you feel your head needs support, place a rolled-up towel under it to raise it just a bit. Make sure that you are not curled up in the fetal position.

2
Reach your right arm in front of you and, keeping it a few inches from the floor, trace a half circle over your head.

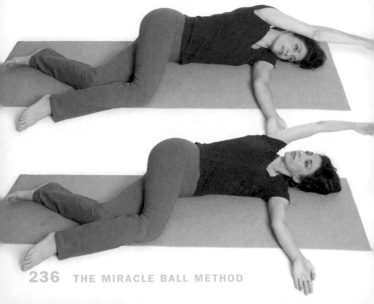

Do not go past the point where you cannot move easily.

3 When you can comfortably go no further, let your rib cage give in to gravity and your arm fall to the floor.

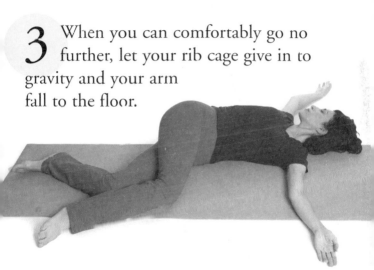

Stay in this position as long as you feel you can give in to your body's weight. Do not stay in the position past the point where it is comfortable. Eventually your shoulder will rest closer to the floor.

4 Slowly roll back onto your left side, tracing the hand just as you did in step 2, but in the opposite direction.

Take notice of your body. Does more of it rest on the floor than when you started? If you used a towel to support your head, are you able to comfortably remove it?

5 Repeat steps 1–4 three times.

When you are finished, roll onto your back and compare the left and right sides of your body. Is the right side closer to the floor? Make the "S" sound as you breathe, and rest here for a few minutes.

6 Repeat steps 1–5 on the opposite side of your body.

CHAPTER EIGHT

Ribs on the Ball

Most of us have absolutely no awareness of the muscles around the rib cage. We don't target them with exercise, perhaps because we don't look in the mirror and think, "Wow, my rib cage is getting thick. I'd better do something about it!" We leave these observations to the usual areas of hips, thighs, and stomach. Because of this lack of awareness, the rib cage is usually very tight.

A complicating factor in a tight rib cage is shallow breathing. As we discussed in How to Breathe (page 57), if you don't breathe fully, the muscles around your ribs become stiff, and when the muscles are stiff, it becomes even more difficult to breathe fully. It's a vicious circle. Tightness in the ribs can contribute to middle back pain, since fully half the vertebrae of the spine are connected to the rib cage. A tight rib cage causes problems with your figure as well. If your rib cage is not supple, it tends to slump into your lower back, which causes your abdominal muscles to protrude. Bye-bye waistline.

After doing Ribs on the Ball, you'll feel as if you've taken off a tight elastic bandage that you've been wearing around your ribs for years. As a bonus, you're likely to get your waistline back. In addition to relief of some back pain, you may notice symptoms of depression and anxiety easing. Shallow breathing is closely linked to these conditions, so loosening the binding on your lungs can be a help.

Exercise One

- **Ribs on the Ball**
- **relieves mid-back pain, shoulder tension; reshapes waistline**

This pose may seem awkward at first. Most people's muscles are so tense that their rib cage feels as if it's one solid piece of plywood. In fact, it is incredibly flexible. Think of it like a new pair of leather shoes—stiff and ungiving at first; flexible after a few sessions of breaking in. This exercise is designed to "break in" your stiff rib cage. If you are so stiff that you feel you are straining your neck, support it on a small pillow or a rolled-up towel. You should feel the weight of your rib cage in this exercise, not your neck and head.

The hardest part of Ribs on the Ball is remembering to give in. Position the ball so that you can let go and breathe. Don't lock your muscles. You need to have the sense that you are draping your limp body over the ball. You may need to move the ball several times under your ribs until you find a place that is comfortable enough to enable you to let go and breathe.

1 Begin by lying on your side on the floor.

Choose the side that you can roll onto the most comfortably. Bend your knees a little bit, but try not to curl into the fetal position. Imagine that you have a mirror on the ceiling and when you look up, you can see that from your hips to the top of your head you form a nice long line, not a tight curve.

2 Place the ball under the side of your ribs.

Roll back a little, then roll your rib cage up onto the ball. Focus on using your rib cage itself to get on and off the ball, and not compensating with muscles from other parts of your body such as your head. If you don't like the feeling of the ball in the middle of your rib cage, try moving it closer to your waistline or your armpit. Give in to the weight of your body. If you can, stay on the ball for 2 to 3 minutes.

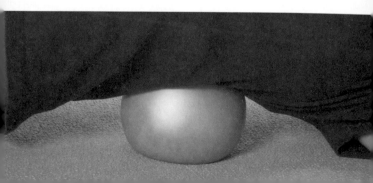

3 Remember to breathe.

This may feel awkward at first, but it is very important for relaxing your muscles and feeling more comfortable. If you hold your breath, your muscles will tighten. By breathing, you will relax the muscles and feel more comfortable.

4 Take the ball away by rolling slightly backward. Let your rib cage sink into the floor.

Is breathing easier? Do you feel that more of your rib cage is pressing into the floor?

5 Repeat going on and off the ball 2 to 3 times on one side.

6 Roll over and do the exercise on your other side.

Exercise Two

- **Ribs on the Ball Facing Up**
- relieves mid-back pain, shoulder tension; realigns spine; reduces stress

1 Lie down on the floor with your knees bent, feet resting flat on the floor.

2 Roll to the side and place a ball beneath the middle of your back.

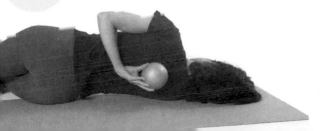

251

3 Roll up onto the ball.

At this point, if you feel
you need back support,
keep your knees
bent; otherwise
slide your feet along the floor until your
legs are straight. Remember to breathe.
If you find that your head and neck are
uncomfortable in this position, place the
second ball under either one.

4 Take the ball away by rolling slightly to
the side and quickly removing the ball.

Whole Body Move

- **Rib Cage Arch**
- reshapes body; improves posture and breathing

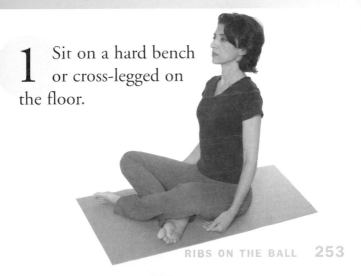

1 Sit on a hard bench or cross-legged on the floor.

2 Keeping your sit bones (the pointy bones at the base of your pelvis) on the bench or floor, arch your rib cage to one side.

Stay in position for a few seconds, letting yourself breathe and feeling the gravity of the movement. Remember to breathe. You must keep your pelvis anchored to the bench or floor in order to feel a stretch along your ribs and waist.

3 Slowly straighten your spine and ribs.

Notice your breathing for a few seconds. Feel the difference between your two sides. Does the side you just stretched feel looser?

4 Repeat the arch on the same side.

Notice that the upper arm hangs from the shoulder. Your palm and wrist should rest on the bench or floor. Your arm should not be outstretched, pulling you away from your sit bones. It should be dropped, limp, right along your side. Feel the shape your entire backbone is forming; make sure you are not curling your head and neck forward but are truly arching your side, with your ear, shoulder, and hip aligned. Feel the stretch along the side of your body. Stay for a few seconds. Breathe.

5 Repeat one more time on the same side. Then repeat the movement 3 times in the opposite direction. When you finish, you should be sitting up straight, with your torso centered over your sit bones.

6 If the preceding steps were comfortable for you, then you may try this. If you feel you are very stiff, then do not attempt it. Reaching your opposite arm over and into the arch with you, repeat the entire exercise 3 times on each side.

If you are arching right, raise your left arm; arching left, raise your right arm. Do this gently; let your rib cage bend just like a waterfall going up and over, a half circle. Reach the hand, notice both sit bones on the floor. Let your head and neck give. Breathe. Stay there for a few seconds, and then return to sitting.

- **Rib Cage Walk**
- **tones entire torso; lengthens lower back muscles; restores energy**

1 Sit cross-legged on the floor and bend forward from your hip joint until your elbows touch the floor.

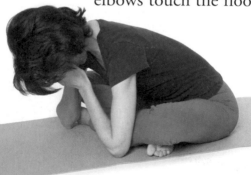

If you can't sit cross-legged, sit as you normally would on a hard bench, with another chair or bench of the same height in front of you. It is important that the bend is initiated from the hip joints. You should be feeling the give there, not in the middle of your back.

2 Rest your face in your hands and "walk" your elbows along the floor. (If you are using a bench to sit on, walk your elbows along the surface of

the bench or chair that you've pulled in front of you.)

Use the muscles surrounding your ribs and along your back to walk your elbows away from you as far as is comfortable without strain. Stay stretched out for 10 to 15 seconds. Sense the lifting and lengthening of your rib cage. Notice your breathing; make the "S" sound.

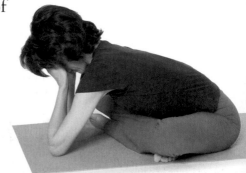

3 Return to sitting, and then repeat the movement 3 times, staying stretched out for the last repetition.

Feel the weight of your body hanging forward onto your elbows.

4 Open up one elbow. Feel the stretch along the side of your body and then bring the elbow back down.

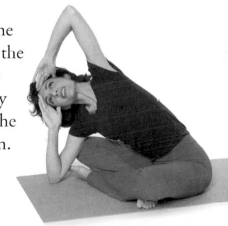

Don't muscle the elbow open from the shoulder; make your rib cage initiate the movement. It's better to make a much smaller motion and feel it coming from the center of your body, than to make a larger motion that originates in your shoulder.

5 Open up the other elbow. Stretch along that side and bring the elbow back down.

Remember to breathe.

6 Repeat steps 4 and 5, alternating sides, 3 times.

CHAPTER NINE

Shoulders on the Ball

In an ideal world, we would stand upright effortlessly. We would be supported by the muscles surrounding our flexible hip joints, and our shoulders would rest effortlessly on our torsos. In reality, most of us use our shoulders to hold ourselves up all day long. We fight gravity by shrugging our shoulders up to our ears, which takes enormous effort and results in tired muscles and stiff joints.

When the shoulder joint becomes stiff, we may suffer pain in our backs or parts of our arms—the elbows, the hands, the fingers. These body parts can only be as agile as the shoulders are relaxed. This chapter offers you very simple shoulder exercises that will help relieve pain emanating from your shoulders by loosening the tension around the shoulder joints and upper spine. Sufferers of carpal tunnel syndrome, frozen shoulder, and tennis elbow will all benefit from easing shoulder tension.

Exercise One

- **Shoulders on the Ball**
- **relieves neck and shoulder tension; eases tension headaches; promotes relaxation**

1 Lie down on an exercise mat or the floor, bend your knees, and rest your feet flat on the floor.

Take note of how you are breathing and which parts of your shoulders are resting on the floor. Your hands should be palms up; this helps ease the shoulders back toward the floor.

2 Take a ball in each hand. Place one ball under each shoulder blade.

Do this by rolling onto your right side, reaching over with your right hand and placing the ball in back of your left shoulder.

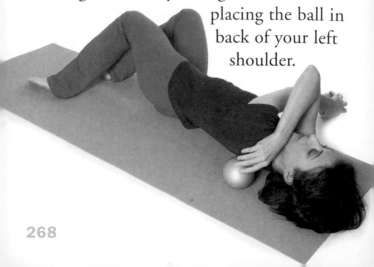

Then
roll up
onto that ball,
reach your left hand
over, and place the other
ball under your right shoulder.
Use your legs to gently roll yourself up
or down a tad to move the balls to a
comfortable spot. Note that placing the
balls higher up the back is easier to do and
more comfortable than putting them lower.

If you feel neck pain, roll up a towel and support your

head with it. Try to wean yourself from the towel eventually. It is natural and healthy for your neck to bend this way; you may not be used to it yet.

Alternate Move:

   You can place the ball from your right hand under your right shoulder blade, roll up onto that ball, and then place the ball from your left hand under your left shoulder blade. Again, shimmy up or down to get the balls to a comfortable spot on your back.

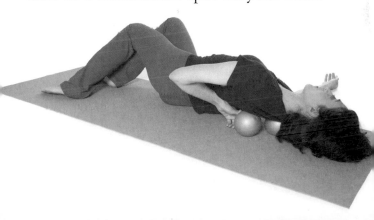

3 Once you feel comfortable with the balls under your shoulders, stretch your legs out.

Rest on the balls for 2 to 3 minutes and let gravity draw you into them. Breathe.

4 With your palms up, move your arms out to the side, to shoulder level.

Stay on the balls, breathing, for 2 to 3 minutes. Sense whether one arm or shoulder gives in to the ball more than the other does.

5 Remove the balls, one at a time, easing your shoulders down to the floor.

Compare the way your shoulders rest on the floor now with the way they rested before you started. Breathe.

6 Repeat the series 3 times.

Exercise Two

- **Shoulders on the Ball with Shrug and Crossed Arms**
- relieves frozen shoulders and carpal tunne syndrome; increases flexibility in shoulde

1 Place two balls under your shoulders as for Shoulders on the Ball (page 267).

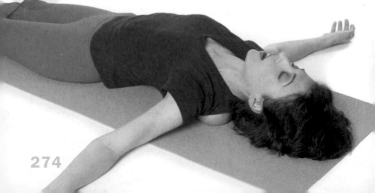

2 Very, very slowly, "shrug" both shoulders up toward your ears slightly and then release them back down. Repeat 3 times.

Be mindful not to lose the feeling of letting your weight sink into the balls. You're just lightly "shrugging"—raising your shoulders slightly toward your ears and then letting them back down.

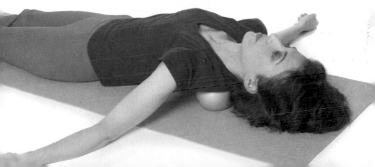

3 Lift your hands toward the ceiling, then cross your arms.

The right hand falls across to your left side, the left hand falls across to your right side. Rest in this position for 30 seconds or longer.

4 Raise your arms over your head and let them rest on the floor, uncrossing them as you bring them into place.

Do this by unfurling your arms with roughly the same movement you would use to take off a T-shirt.

Rest in this new position for about 30 seconds, with your arms extended and your hands reaching away from your shoulders. If they are not comfortable, move them apart until they rest easily and comfortably above your head. Let your back arch if it wants to. Feel this through the rest of your body, and then bring your arms down, extended, to shoulder level. Repeat 1 time, slowly, taking notice of how your body gives in. Finish with your hands resting loosely by your sides.

5 Now shimmy down a little bit, using your hips and feet to move you downward. The balls are positioned 1 to 2 inches higher up your back, toward the back of your neck.

6 Rest on the balls in this new position. As you did in step 3, reach your arms toward the ceiling, then let them cross over your chest.

Exhale. Feel the weight. Notice that the space between your shoulder blades is starting to widen. Are you getting a better sense of the muscles being used?

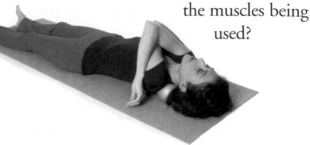

7 Stretch your arms overhead as you did in steps 3 and 4, then bring them to rest at your sides.

8 Shimmy down one more time. The balls should be as far up your body as they can be without slipping out of place. Rest here.

You shouldn't need anything under your neck or head at this point because the balls are up so high that very little of your back is lifted. The muscles that are resting on the ball are usually very tense, and they need some time to let go. Breathe and remain in this position for 3 to 5 minutes.

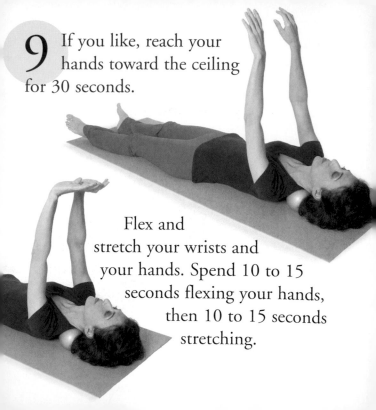

9 If you like, reach your hands toward the ceiling for 30 seconds.

Flex and stretch your wrists and your hands. Spend 10 to 15 seconds flexing your hands, then 10 to 15 seconds stretching.

10 Bring your arms across your chest as before and let them relax there.

Give in to gravity and remember to breathe.

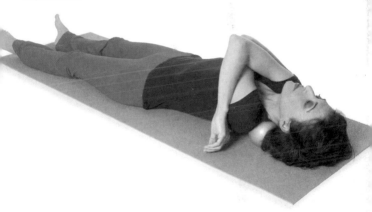

11 Remove the balls, one at a time.

Take note of your body. What parts of it are making contact with the floor? Roll your head and neck slowly from side to side a few times. Does your chest feel looser?

- **Kneeling Spider Walk**
- stretches back muscles; relieves neck and shoulder tension; reshapes entire body

1 Kneel on the floor.

If you can't kneel comfortably, sit as you normally would on a hard bench, with another chair or bench in front of you.

2 Creep your fingertips forward along the floor or chair a few inches at a time, first with one hand and then the other. Make sure you are letting your shoulders move as your hands pull you forward. Do not resist the motion. Feel the movement throughout your back. It should take you 8 to 10 small steps to do this.

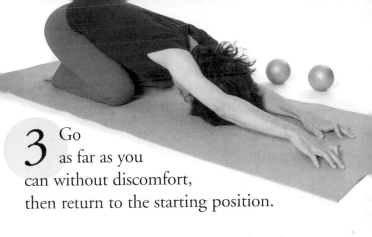

3 Go as far as you can without discomfort, then return to the starting position.

Has your body changed after this lengthening? Most people notice their shoulders are farther from their ears, and that they are at ease, with the rest of the body supporting them.

Index

About the Author

Elaine Petrone developed her method of stress and pain reduction from her own experiences with chronic pain. She has written for and has been featured in a host of magazines, including *Fitness, Vogue, Woman's Day, Glamour, Redbook, Self, American Spa, Elle, Town & Country,* and *Harper's Bazaar*. Ms. Petrone teaches her method in hospitals, and is developing a national certification program for instructors. She can be reached at: elaine@elainepetrone.com.

Elaine Petrone is available for select speaking engagements. Please contact speakersbureau@workman.com.

Acknowledgments

This book has developed from a journey I began more than 25 years ago, with the help of many people. Elaine Summers, Elsa Gindler, Mabel Todd, and others—I owe them all deep gratitude.

Thanks to Elliot Zelevansky for all his encouragement. Thanks to Jane Ubell Meyer for her support and introducing me to my agent Bob Silverstein. Bob is not just an agent but someone who understands my message and knew I needed a special publisher to accomplish it.

Thanks to the people at Workman Publishing—Peter Workman, Suzie Bolotin, Jennifer Griffin, Cindy Schoen, Paul Hanson, Elizabeth Johnsboen, Marta Jaremko, and Elizabeth Gaynor—for tackling a complicated project.

Thanks to my children, John, Lucas, and Rose who many times have had to explain to their friends why there were hundreds of balls of varying sizes all over the house and why their mom was always lying on the floor. They have forced me to grow in ways I never imagined. They are my reason for being.

Finally, thanks to my students, who have allowed me to teach and learn from them. My hope is that everyone who tries the Miracle Ball Method will discover the unrealized potential their bodies have to heal and thrive.

—ELAINE PETRONE